The Air Fryer Beginners' Cooking Guide

A Complete Collection of Meat Recipes to Start Your air Fryer Diet and Boost Your Taste

Franck McMillan

TABLE OF CONTENT

medical or professional advice. The content within this book has been derived from various sources. Please consult a licensed professional before attempting any techniques outlined in this book.

By reading this document, the reader agrees that under no circumstances is the author responsible for any losses, direct or indirect, which are incurred as a result of the use of information contained within this document, including, but not limited to, — errors, omissions, or inaccuracies.

Cajun Cheese Sticks

Preparation Time:5 Minutes

Cooking Time: 15 Minutes

Servings: 4

Ingredients:

- 1/2 cup all-purpose flour
- Two eggs
- 1/2 cup parmesan cheese, grated
- One tablespoon Cajun seasonings
- Eight cheese sticks, kid-friendly

Directions:

1. To begin, set up your breading station. Place the all-purpose flour in a dish. In a separate dish, whisk the eggs.
2. Finally, mix the parmesan cheese and Cajun seasoning in a third dish.
3. Start by dredging the cheese sticks in the flour; then, dip them into the egg. Press the cheese sticks into the parmesan mixture, coating evenly.
4. Place the breaded cheese sticks in the lightly greased Air Fryer basket. Cook with settings at 380 degrees F for 6 minutes.

5. Serve with ketchup and enjoy!

Nutrition: Calories 372 Fat 27g Carbs 15g Protein 28g Sugar 8g

Classic Deviled Eggs

Preparation Time:5 Minutes

Cooking Time: 20 Minutes

Servings: 3

Ingredients:

- Five eggs
- Two tablespoons mayonnaise
- Two tablespoons sweet pickle relish
- Sea salt, to taste
- 1/2 teaspoon mixed peppercorns, crushed

Directions:

1. Put the wire rack in the Air Fryer basket; lower the eggs onto the wire rack.
2. Cook utilizing 270 degrees F for 15 minutes.
3. Handover them to an ice-cold water bath to stop the cooking
4. Peel the eggs underneath cold running water; slice them into halves.
5. Puree the egg yolks with the mayo, sweet pickle relish, salt; spoon yolk mixture into egg whites. Assemble on a nice serving

platter and garnish with the mixed peppercorns. Bon appétit!

Nutrition: Calories 261 Fat 12g Carbs 5g Protein 15g Sugar 1g

Barbecue Little Smokies

Preparation Time:5 Minutes

Cooking Time: 20 Minutes

Servings: 6

Ingredients:
- 1-pound beef cocktail wieners
- 10 ounces barbecue sauce

Directions:
1. Twitch by preheating your Air Fryer to 380 degrees F.
2. Prick holes into your sausages using a fork and transfer them to the baking pan.
3. Cook for 13 minutes. Spoon the barbecue sauce into the pan and cook an additional 2 minutes.
4. Serve with toothpicks. Bon appétit!

Nutrition: Calories 182 Fat 6g Carbs 12g Protein 19g Sugar 17g

Paprika Potato Chips

Preparation Time: 5 Minutes

Cooking Time: 45 Minutes

Servings: 3

Ingredients:

- Three potatoes, thinly sliced
- One teaspoon sea salt
- One teaspoon garlic powder
- One teaspoon paprika
- 1/4 cup ketchup

Directions:

1. Add the sliced potatoes to a bowl with salted water. Let them soak for 30 minutes. Drain and rinse your potatoes.
2. Pat dry and toss with salt.
3. Cook in the preheated Air Fryer set at 400 degrees F for 15 minutes, occasionally shaking the basket.
4. Work in batches. Toss with the garlic powder and paprika. Serve with ketchup. Enjoy!

Nutrition: Calories 190 Fat 3g Carbs 48g Protein 7g Sugar 1g

Cheddar Dip

Preparation Time:5 Minutes

Cooking Time: 15 Minutes

Servings: 6

Ingredients:

- 8 oz. cheddar cheese; grated
- 12 oz. coconut cream
- 2 tsp. hot sauce

Directions:

1. In a ramekin, mix the cream with hot sauce and cheese and whisk.
2. Put the ramekin in the fryer and cook at 390°F for 12 minutes. Whisk, divide into bowls, and serve as a dip

Nutrition: Calories: 170 Fat: 9g Fiber: 2g Carbs: 4g Protein: 12g

Coated Avocado Tacos

Preparation Time:10 Minutes

Cooking Time: 20 Minutes

Servings: 12

Ingredients:

- 1 avocado
- Tortillas and toppings
- ½ cup panko breadcrumbs
- 1 egg
- Salt

Directions:

- Scoop out the meat from each avocado shell and slice them into wedges.
- Beat the egg in a shallow bowl and put the breadcrumbs in another bowl.
- Dip the avocado wedges in the beaten egg and coat with breadcrumbs. Sprinkle them with a bit of salt. Arrange them in the cooking basket in a single layer.
- Cook for 15 minutes at 392 degrees. Shake the basket halfway through the cooking process.

- Put the cooked avocado wedges in tortillas and add your preferred toppings.

Nutrition: Calories: 179 Fat: 07g Carbs: 229g Protein: 94g

Roasted Corn with Butter and Lime

Preparation Time:2 Minutes

Cooking Time: 20 Minutes

Servings: 4

Ingredients:

- 4 corns
- ½ tsp. Pepper
- 1 tsp. Lime juice
- 1 tbsp. Chopped parsley
- 1 tbsp. Butter
- ¼ tsp. Salt

Directions:

1. Preheat air fryer to a temperature of 400°f.
2. Remove husk and transfer corns into air fryer and cook for 20 minutes.
3. After every 5 minutes shake the fryer basket.
4. When done rub butter. Sprinkle parsley, pepper, and salt. Drizzle lime juice on top. Serve!

Nutrition: Calories: 114 Protein: 4g Fat: 26g Carbs:

124g

Batter-Fried Scallions

Preparation Time:5 Minutes

Cooking Time: 5 Minutes

Servings: 4

Ingredients:

- Trimmed scallion bunches,
- White wine, 1 cup
- Salt, 1 tsp.
- Flour, 1 cup
- Black pepper, 1 tsp

Directions:

1. Set the air fryer to heat up to 390F. Using a bowl, add and mix the white wine, flour and stir until it gets smooth. Add the salt, the black pepper and mix again. Dip each scallion into the flour mixture until it is properly covered and remove any excess batter. Grease your air fryer basket with nonstick cooking spray and add the scallions. At this point, you may need to work in batches.
2. Leave the scallions to cook for 5 minutes or until it has a golden-brown color and crispy

texture, while still shaking it after every 2 minutes. Carefully remove it from your air fryer and check if it's properly done. Then allow it to cool before serving. Serve and enjoy.

Nutrition: Calories: 179 Fat: 07g Carbs: 229g Protein: 94g

Heirloom Tomato with Baked Feta

Preparation Time: 20 Minutes

Cooking Time: 14 Minutes

Servings: 4

Ingredients:

- 8 oz. Feta cheese
- Salt
- 2 heirloom tomatoes
- ½ cup sliced red onions
- 1 tbsp. Olive oil
- For the basil pesto
- ½ cup grated parmesan cheese
- Salt
- ½ cup olive oil
- 3 tbsps. Toasted pine nuts
- ½ cup chopped basil
- 1 garlic clove
- ½ cup chopped parsley

Directions:

1. Directions: are the pesto.

2. Put the toasted pine nuts, garlic, salt, basil, and parmesan in a food processor. Process until combined.
3. Gradually add oil as you mix. Process until everything is blended.
4. Transfer to a bowl and cover. Refrigerate until ready to use.
5. Slice the feta and tomato into round slices with half an inch thickness. Use paper towels to pat them dry.
6. Spread a tbsp. Of pesto on top of each tomato slice.
7. Top with a slice of feta.
8. In a small bowl, mix a tbsp. Of olive oil and red onions.
9. Scoop the mixture on top of the feta layer. Arrange them in the cooking basket. Cook for 14 minutes at 390 f.
10. Transfer to a platter and add a tbsp. Of basil pesto on top of each. Sprinkle them with a bit of salt before serving.

Nutrition: Calories: 493 Fat: 423g Carbs: 61g Protein: 169g

Crispy Potato Skins

Preparation Time: 5 Minutes

Cooking Time: 55 Minutes

Servings: 2

Ingredients:

1. 2 Yukon gold potatoes
2. ¼ tsp. Sea salt
3. ½ tsp. Olive oil
4. 2 minced green onions, 4 bacon strips
5. ¼ cup shredded cheddar cheese, 1/3 cup sour cream

Directions:

1. Rinse and scrub the potatoes until clean. Rub with oil and sprinkle with salt. Put them in the cooking basket. Cook for 35 minutes at 400 degrees. Transfer the cooked potatoes to a platter. Put the bacon strip in the cooking basket. Cook for 5 minutes at 400 f.
2. Move to a plate and leave to cool. Crumble into bits.
3. Slice the potatoes in half.

4. Scoop out most of the meat. Arrange the potato skins with the skin facing side up in the cooking basket. Spray them with oil. Cook for 3 minutes at 400 f. Flip the potato skins. Fill each piece with cheese and crumbled bacon. Continue cooking for 2 more minutes. Transfer to a platter. Add a bit of sour cream on top. Sprinkle with minced onion and serve while warm.

Nutrition: Calories: 483 Fat: 73g Carbs: 98g Protein: 152g

Beets and Carrots

Preparation Time:1 Minutes

Cooking Time: 12 Minutes

Servings: 4

Ingredients:

- 4 carrots whole
- 4 sliced young beetroots
- ¼ tsp. Black pepper
- 1 tsp. Olive oil
- ¼ tsp. Salt
- 1 tbsps. Lemon juice

Directions:

1. Preheat air fryer to a temperature of 400°f (200°c.
2. Transfer beetroots and carrots to air fryer basket and sprinkle salt and pepper. Drizzle olive oil and toss to combine.
3. Leave to cook for 12 minutes. Shake the basket of fryer after halftime. Remove from the air fryer and drizzle lemon juice. Serve and enjoy!

Nutrition: Calories: 71 Protein: 92g Fat: 43g Carbs: 106g

Broccoli Crisps

Preparation Time: 10 Minutes

Cooking Time: 12 Minutes

Servings: 4

Ingredients:

- Large chopped broccoli head,
- Salt, 1 tsp.
- Olive oil, 2 tbsps.
- Black pepper, 1 tsp.

Directions:

1. Set the air fryer to heat up to 3600f.
2. Using a bowl, add and toss the broccoli florets with olive oil, salt, and black pepper.
3. Add the broccoli florets and cook it for 12 minutes, then shake after 6 minutes.
4. Carefully remove it from your air fryer and allow it to cool off.
5. Serve and enjoy!

Nutrition: Calories: 120 Fat: 19g Protein: 5g Carbs: 3g

Maple Syrup Bacon

Preparation Time:5 Minutes

Cooking Time: 10 Minutes

Servings: 2

Ingredients:

- Maple syrup.
- Thick bacon slices, 1

Directions:

1. Preheat your air fryer to 400°f.
2. Place the bacon on the flat surface and brush with the maple syrup.
3. Move to the air fryer to cook for 10 minutes.
4. Serve and enjoy!

Nutrition: Calories: 91 Carbs: 0g Protein: 8g Fat: 2g

Low-Carb Pizza Crust

Preparation Time: 10 Minutes

Cooking Time: 20 Minutes

Servings: 4

Ingredients:

- 1 tbsp. full-fat cream cheese
- ½ cup whole-milk mozzarella cheese, shredded
- 2 tbsp. flour
- 1 egg white

Directions:

1. Directions: are the cream cheese, mozzarella, and flour in a microwaveable bowl and heat in the microwave for half a minute. Mix well to create a smooth consistency. Add in the egg white and stir to form a soft ball of dough.
2. With slightly wet hands, press the dough into a pizza crust about six inches in diameter.
3. Arrange sheet of parchment paper in the bottom of your fryer and lay the crust on top. Cook for ten minutes at 350degreesF,

turning the crust over halfway through the cooking Time.

4. Top the pizza base with the toppings of your choice and enjoy!

Nutrition: Calories: 260 Fat: 21g Carbs: 6g Protein: 9g

Colby Potato Patties

Preparation Time:5 Minutes

Cooking Time: 15 Minutes

Servings: 8

Ingredients:

- 2 lb. white potatoes, peeled and grated
- ½ cup scallions, finely chopped
- ½ tsp. freshly ground black pepper
- 1tbsp. fine sea salt
- ½ tsp. hot paprika
- 2 cups Colby cheese, shredded
- ¼ cup canola oil
- 1 cup crushed crackers

Directions:

1. Boil the potatoes until soft. Dry them off and peel them before mashing thoroughly, leaving no lumps.
2. Combine the mashed potatoes with scallions, pepper, salt, paprika, and cheese.
3. Shape mixture into balls with your hands and press with your palm to flatten them into patties.

4. In shallow dish, combine the canola oil and crushed crackers. Coat the patties in the crumb mixture.
5. Cook the patties at 360degreesF for about 10 minutes, in multiple batches if necessary.
6. Serve with tabasco mayo or the sauce of your choice.

Nutrition: Calories: 130 Fat: 7g Carbs: 17g Protein: 1g

Turkey Garlic Potatoes

Preparation Time:10 Minutes

Cooking Time: 45 Minutes

Servings: 2

Ingredients:

- unsmoked turkey strips
- small potatoes
- 1 tsp. garlic, minced
- 2 tsp. olive oil
- Salt to taste
- Pepper to taste

Directions:

1. Peel the potatoes and cube them finely.
2. Coat in 1 teaspoon of oil and cook in the Air Fryer for 10 minutes at 350degreesF.
3. In separate bowl, slice the turkey finely and combine with the garlic, oil, salt and pepper. Pour the potatoes into the bowl and mix well.
4. Lay the mixture on some silver aluminum foil, transfer to the fryer and cook for about 10 minutes.
5. Serve with raita.

Nutrition: Calories: 210 Fat: 4g Carbs: 22g Protein: 22g

Creamy Scrambled Eggs

Preparation Time:5 Minutes

Cooking Time: 15 Minutes

Servings: 2

Ingredients:

- 2 tbsp. olive oil, melted
- eggs, whisked
- oz. fresh spinach, chopped
- 1 medium-sized tomato, chopped
- 1 tsp. fresh lemon juice
- ½ tsp. coarse salt
- ½ tsp. ground black pepper
- ½ cup of fresh basil, roughly chopped

Directions:

1. Grease the Air Fryer baking pan with the oil, tilting it to spread the oil around. Pre-heat the fryer at 280degreesF.
2. Mix the remaining ingredients, apart from the basil leaves, whisking well until everything is completely combined.
3. Cook in the fryer for 8 - 12 minutes.
4. Top with fresh basil leaves before serving with little sour cream if desired.

Nutrition: Calories: 140 Fat: 10g Carbs: 2g Protein: 12g

Bacon-Wrapped Onion Rings

Preparation Time:10 Minutes

Cooking Time: 15 Minutes

Servings: 8

Ingredients:

- 1 large onion, peeled
- slices sugar-free bacon
- 1 tbsp. sriracha

Directions:

1. Chop up the onion into slices a quarter-inch thick. Gently pull apart the rings. Take a slice of bacon and wrap it around an onion ring. Repeat with the rest of the ingredients.
2. Place each onion ring in your fryer.
3. Cut the onion rings at 350degreesF for ten minutes, turning them halfway through to ensure the bacon crisps up.
4. Serve hot with the sriracha.

Nutrition: Calories: 280 Fat: 19g Carbs: 25g Protein: 3g

Grilled Cheese

Preparation Time:5 Minutes

Cooking Time: 25 Minutes

Servings: 2

Ingredients:

- 4 slices of bread
- ½ cup sharp cheddar cheese
- ¼ cup butter, melted

Directions:

1. Pre-heat the Air Fryer at 360degreesF.
2. Put cheese and butter in separate bowls.
3. Apply the butter to each side of the bread slices with a brush.
4. Spread the cheese across two of the slices of bread and make two sandwiches. Transfer both to the fryer.
5. Cook for 5 – 7 minutes or until a golden-brown color is achieved and the cheese is melted.

Nutrition: Calories: 170 Fat: 8g Carbs: 17g Protein: 5g

Peppered Puff Pastry

Preparation Time:10 Minutes

Cooking Time: 25 Minutes

Servings: 4

Ingredients:

- 1 ½ tbsp. sesame oil
- 1 cup white mushrooms, sliced
- 2 cloves garlic, minced
- 1 bell pepper, seeded and chopped
- ¼ tsp. sea salt
- ¼ tsp. dried rosemary
- ½ tsp. ground black pepper, or more to taste
- oz. puff pastry sheets
- ½ cup crème fraiche
- 1 egg, well whisked
- ½ cup parmesan cheese, preferably freshly grated

Directions:

1. Pre-heat your Air Fryer to 400degreesF.
2. Heat the sesame oil over moderate temperature and fry the mushrooms, garlic, and pepper until soft and fragrant.

3. Sprinkle on the salt, rosemary, and pepper.
4. In the meantime, unroll the puff pastry and slice it into 4-inch squares.
5. Spread the crème fraiche across each square.
6. Spoon equal amounts of the vegetables into the puff pastry squares. Enclose each square around the filling in triangle shape, pressing the edges with your fingertips.
7. Brush each triangle with some whisked egg and cover with grated Parmesan.
8. Cook for 22-25 minutes.

Nutrition: Calories: 259 Fat: 18g Carbs: 21g Protein: 3g

Horseradish Mayo & Gorgonzola Mushrooms

Preparation Time:10 Minutes

Cooking Time: 15 Minutes

Servings: 5

Ingredients:

- ½ cup of breadcrumbs
- 2 cloves garlic, pressed
- 2 tbsp. fresh coriander, chopped
- 1/3 tsp. kosher salt
- ½ tsp. crushed red pepper flakes
- 1 ½ tbsp. olive oil
- 2 medium-sized mushrooms, stems removed
- ½ cup Gorgonzola cheese, grated
- ¼ cup low-fat mayonnaise
- 1 tsp. horseradish, well-drained
- 1 tbsp. fresh parsley, finely chopped

Directions:

1. Combine the breadcrumbs together with the garlic, coriander, salt, red pepper, and the olive oil.

2. Take equal-sized amounts of the bread crumb mixture and use them to stuff the mushroom caps. Add the grated Gorgonzola on top of each.
3. Put the mushrooms in the Air Fryer grill pan and transfer to the fryer.
4. Grill them at 380degreesF for 8-12 minutes, ensuring the stuffing is warm throughout.
5. In the meantime, Directions: are the horseradish mayo. Mix together the mayonnaise, horseradish and parsley.
6. When the mushrooms are ready, serve with the mayo.

Nutrition: Calories: 140 Fat: 13g Carbs: 6g Protein: 0g

Crumbed Beans

Preparation Time: 5 Minutes

Cooking Time: 10 Minutes

Servings: 4

Ingredients:

- ½ cup flour
- 1 tsp. smoky chipotle powder
- ½ tsp. ground black pepper
- 1 tsp. sea salt flakes
- 2 eggs, beaten
- ½ cup crushed saltines
- 20 oz. wax beans

Directions:

1. Combine the flour, chipotle powder, black pepper, and salt in a bowl. Put the eggs in second bowl. Place the crushed saltines in third bowl.
2. Wash the beans with cold water and discard any tough strings.
3. Coat the beans with the flour mixture, before dipping them into the beaten egg. Lastly cover them with the crushed saltines.

4. Spritz the beans with cooking spray.

5. Air-fry at 360degreesF for 4 minutes. Give the cooking basket a good shake and continue to cook for 3 minutes. Serve hot.

Nutrition: Calories: 200 Fat: 8g Carbs: 27g Protein: 4g

CROUTONS

Preparation Time:5 Minutes

Cooking Time: 10 Minutes

Servings: 4

Ingredients:

- 2 slices friendly bread
- 1 tbsp. olive oil

Directions:

1. Cut the slices of bread into medium-size chunks.
2. Coat the inside of the Air Fryer with the oil. Set it to 390degreesF and allow it to heat up.
3. Place the chunks inside and shallow fry for at least 8 minutes.
4. Serve with hot soup.

Nutrition: Calories: 186 Fat: 7g Carbs: 25g Protein: 4g

Cheese Lings

Preparation Time: 5 Minutes

Cooking Time: 25 Minutes

Servings: 6

Ingredients:

- 1 cup flour
- small cubes cheese, grated
- ¼ tsp. chili powder
- 1 tsp. butter
- Salt to taste
- 1 tsp. baking powder

Directions:

1. Put all Ingredients: to form a dough, along with a small amount water as necessary.
2. Divide the dough into equal portions and roll each one into a ball.
3. Pre-heat Air Fryer at 360degreesF.
4. Transfer the balls to the fryer and air fry for 5 minutes, stirring periodically.

Nutrition: Calories: 489 Fat: 20g Carbs: 69g Protein: 8g

Sweet Potato Wedges

Preparation Time:10 Minutes

Cooking Time: 20 Minutes

Servings: 4

Ingredients:

- 2 sweet potatoes, sliced into wedges
- 1 tablespoon vegetable oil
- 1 teaspoon smoked paprika
- 1 tablespoon honey
- Salt and pepper to taste

Directions:

1. Add air fryer basket to your Power XL Grill.
2. Choose air fry setting.
3. Preheat at 390 degrees for 25 minutes.
4. Add sweet potato wedges to the basket.
5. Cook for 10 minutes.
6. Stir and cook for another 10 minutes.
7. Toss in paprika and honey.
8. Sprinkle with salt and pepper.

Nutrition: Calories – 368 Fat – 24.2g Carbohydrates – 21g Fiber – 4.1g Protein – 17.6g

Spiced Almonds

Preparation Time:5 minutes

Cooking Time: 10 minutes

Servings: 4

Ingredients:

- 1/2 tsp. ground cinnamon
- 1/2 tsp. smoked paprika
- 1 cup almonds - 1 egg white

Directions:

1. Preheat air fryer to 310 F. Grease the air fryer basket with cooking spray. In a bowl, beat the egg white with cinnamon and paprika and stir in almonds.
2. Spread the almonds on the bottom of the frying basket and Air Fry for 12 minutes, shaking once or twice. Remove and sprinkle with sea salt to serve.

Nutrition: Calories: 90 Carbs: 3 g Fat: 2 g Protein: 5 g

Crispy Cauliflower Bites

Preparation Time:5 minutes

Cooking Time: 15 minutes

Servings: 4

Ingredients:

- 1 tbsp. Italian seasoning
- 1 cup flour - 1 cup milk
- 1 egg, beaten
- 1 head cauliflower, cut into florets

Directions:

1. Preheat air fryer to 390 F. Grease the air fryer basket with cooking spray. In a bowl, mix the flour, milk, egg, and Italian seasoning. Coat the cauliflower in the mixture and drain the excess liquid.
2. Place the florets in the frying basket, spray them with cooking spray, and Air Fry for 7 minutes. Shake and continue cooking for another 5 minutes. Allow to cool before serving.

Nutrition: Calories: 70 Carbs: 2 g Fat: 1 g Protein: 3 g

Roasted Coconut Carrots

Preparation Time:5 minutes

Cooking Time: 10 minutes

Servings: 4

Ingredients:

- 1 tbsp. coconut oil, melted
- 1 lb. horse carrots, sliced
- 1/2 tsp. chili powder

Directions:

1. Preheat air fryer to 400 F.
2. In a bowl, mix the carrots with coconut oil, chili powder, salt, and pepper. Place in the air fryer and Air Fry for 7 minutes. Shake the basket and cook for another 5 minutes until golden brown. Serve.

Nutrition: Calories: 80 Carbs: 3 g Fat: 1 g Protein: 4 g

Spicy Grilled Turkey Breast

Preparation Time:10 Minutes

Cooking Time: 40 minutes

Servings: 14

Ingredients:

- 5 lb. turkey breast, bone in
- What you'll need from store cupboard:
- 1 cup low sodium chicken broth
- ¼ cup vinegar
- ¼ cup jalapeno pepper jelly
- 2 tbsp. Splenda brown sugar
- 2 tbsp. olive oil
- 2 tsp cinnamon
- 1 tsp cayenne pepper
- ½ tsp ground mustard
- Nonstick cooking spray

Directions:

1. Heat grill to medium heat. Spray rack with cooking spray. Place a drip pan on the grill for indirect heat.
2. In a small bowl, combine Splenda brown sugar with seasonings.

3. Carefully loosen the skin on the turkey from both sides with your fingers. Spread half the spice mix on the turkey. Secure the skin to the underneath with toothpicks and spread remaining spice mix on the outside.

4. Place the turkey over the drip pan and grill 30 minutes.

5. In a small saucepan, over medium heat, combine broth, vinegar, jelly, and oil. Cook and stir 2 minutes until jelly is completely melted. Reserve ½ cup of the mixture.

6. Baste turkey with some of the jelly mixture. Cook 1-1 ½ hours, basting every 15 minutes, until done, when thermometer reaches 170 degrees.

7. Cover and let rest 10 minutes. Discard the skin. Brush with reserved jelly mixture and slice and serve.

Nutrition: Calories 314 Total Carbs 5g Protein 35g Fat 14g Sugar 5g Fiber 0g

Teriyaki Turkey Bowls

Preparation Time:10 minutes

Cooking Time: 15 minutes

Servings: 4

Ingredients:

- 1 lb. lean ground turkey
- 1 medium head cauliflower, separated into small florets
- What you'll need from store cupboard:
- 1 cup water, divided
- ¼ cup + 1 tbsp. soy sauce
- 2 tbsp. Hoisin sauce
- 2 tbsp. honey
- 1 ½ tbsp. cornstarch
- 1 tsp crushed red pepper flakes
- 1 tsp garlic powder

Directions:

1. In a medium nonstick skillet, cook turkey over med-high heat until brown.
2. In a medium saucepan, combine ¾ cup water, ¼ cup soy sauce, hoisin, pepper flakes, honey, and garlic powder and cook

over medium heat, stirring occasionally, until it starts to bubble.

3. In a small bowl whisk together ¼ cup water and cornstarch and add to the saucepan. Bring mixture to a full boil, stirring occasionally. Once it starts to boil, remove from heat and the turkey. Stir to combine.

4. Place the cauliflower florets in a food processor and pulse until it resembles rice.

5. Spray a nonstick skillet with cooking spray and add the cauliflower and 1 tablespoon soy sauce and cook until cauliflower starts to get soft, about 5-7 minutes.

6. To serve, spoon cauliflower evenly into four bowls, top with turkey mixture and garnish with

Nutrition: Calories 267 Total Carbs 24g Net Carbs 20g Protein 26g Fat 9g Sugar 15g Fiber 4g

Thai Turkey Stir Fry

Preparation Time:5 minutes

Cooking Time: 15 minutes

Servings: 6

Ingredients:

- 1 1/2 lb. lean ground turkey
- 1-2 cups Thai basil, chopped
- 1 onion, cut in slivers
- 1 red bell pepper, cut in thin strips
- 2 tbsp. fresh lime juice
- What you'll need from store cupboard:
- 2-3 large cloves garlic, peeled and sliced
- 1 tbsp. + 1 tsp peanut oil
- 1 tbsp. fish sauce
- 1 tbsp. Sriracha Sauce
- 1 tbsp. soy sauce
- 1 tbsp. honey

Directions:

1. In a small bowl, whisk together lime juice, fish sauce, Sriracha, soy sauce, and honey.
2. Place a large wok or heavy skillet over high heat. Once the pan gets hot, add 1 tablespoon oil and let it get hot. Add garlic

and cook just until fragrant, about 30 seconds. Remove the garlic and discard.

3. Add the onion and bell pepper and cook, stirring frequently 1-2 minutes, or until they start to get soft, transfer to a bowl.

4. Add the remaining oil, if it's needed and cook the turkey, breaking it up as it cooks, until it starts to brown and liquid has evaporated.

5. Add the vegetables back to the pan along with the basil and cook another minute more. Stir in sauce until all ingredients are mixed well. Cook, stirring 2 minutes, or until most of the sauce is absorbed.

Nutrition: Calories 214 Total Carbs 7g Net Carbs 6g Protein 23g Fat 11g Sugar 5g Fiber 1g

Turkey Enchiladas

Preparation Time: 15 minutes

Cooking Time: 35 minutes

Servings: 8

Ingredients:

- 3 cup turkey, cooked and cut in pieces
- 1 onion, diced
- 1 bell pepper, diced
- 1 cup fat free sour cream
- 1 cup reduced fat cheddar cheese, grated
- What you'll need from store cupboard:
- 8 6-inch flour tortillas
- 14 ½ oz. low sodium chicken broth
- ¾ cup salsa
- 3 tbsp. flour
- 2 tsp olive oil
- 1 ¼ tsp coriander
- Nonstick cooking spray

Directions:

1. Spray a large saucepan with cooking spray and heat oil over med-high heat. Add onion and bell pepper and cook until tender.

2. Sprinkle with flour, coriander and pepper and stir until blended. Slowly stir in broth. Bring to a boil and cook, stirring, 2 minutes or until thickened.
3. Remove from heat and stir in sour cream and ¾ cup cheese.
4. Heat oven to 350 degrees. Spray a 13x9-inch pan with cooking spray.
5. In a large bowl, combine turkey, salsa, and 1 cup of cheese mixture. Spoon 1/3 cup mixture down middle of each tortilla and roll up. Place seam side down in dish.
6. Pour remaining cheese mixture over top of enchiladas. Cover and bake 20 minutes. Uncover and sprinkle with remaining cheese. Bake another 5-10 minutes until cheese is melted and starts to brown.

Nutrition: Calories 304 Total Carbs 29g Net Carbs 27g Protein 23g Fat 10g Sugar 5g Fiber 2g

Baked Potatoes with Bacon

Preparation Time:5 minutes

Cooking Time: 30 minutes

Servings: 4

Ingredients:

- 4 potatoes, scrubbed, halved, cut lengthwise
- 1 tbsp. olive oil
- Salt and black pepper to taste
- 4 oz. bacon, chopped

Directions:

1. Preheat air fryer to 390 F. Brush the potatoes with olive oil and season with salt and pepper. Arrange them in the greased frying basket, cut-side down.
2. Bake for 15 minutes, flip them, top with bacon and bake for 12-15 minutes or until potatoes are golden and bacon is crispy. Serve warm.

Nutrition: Calories: 150 Carbs: 9 g Fat: 7 g Protein: 12 g

Walnut & Cheese Filled Mushrooms

Preparation Time: 5 minutes

Cooking Time: 10 minutes

Servings: 4

Ingredients:

- 4 large Portobello mushroom caps
- 1/3 cup walnuts, minced
- 1 tbsp. canola oil
- 1/2 cup mozzarella cheese, shredded
- 2 tbsp. fresh parsley, chopped

Directions:

1. Preheat air fryer to 350 F. Grease the air fryer basket with cooking spray.
2. Rub the mushrooms with canola oil and fill them with mozzarella cheese. Top with minced walnuts and arrange on the bottom of the greased air fryer basket. Bake for 10 minutes or until golden on top. Remove, let cool for a few minutes and sprinkle with freshly chopped parsley to serve.

Nutrition: Calories: 110 Carbs: 6 g Fat: 5 g Protein: 8 g

Air-Fried Chicken Thighs

Preparation Time:5 minutes

Cooking Time: 15 minutes

Servings: 4

Ingredients:

- 1 1/2 lb. chicken thighs
- 2 eggs, lightly beaten
- 1 cup seasoned breadcrumbs
- 1/2 tsp. oregano
- Salt and black pepper, to taste

Directions:

1. Preheat air fryer to 390 F. Season the chicken with oregano, salt, and pepper. In a bowl, add the beaten eggs. In a separate bowl, add the breadcrumbs. Dip chicken thighs in the egg wash, then roll them in the breadcrumbs and press firmly so the breadcrumbs stick well.

2. Spray the chicken with cooking spray and arrange the frying basket in a single layer, skin-side up. Air Fry for 12 minutes, turn the chicken thighs over and continue cooking for 6-8 more minutes. Serve.

Nutrition: Calories: 190 Carbs: 11 g Fat: 8 g Protein: 16 g

Simple Buttered Potatoes

Preparation Time:5 minutes

Cooking Time: 30 minutes

Servings: 4

Ingredients:

- 1-pound potatoes, cut into wedges
- 2 garlic cloves, grated
- 1 tsp. fennel seeds
- 2 tbsp. butter, melted
- Salt and black pepper to taste

Directions:

1. In a bowl, mix the potatoes, butter, garlic, fennel seeds, salt, and black pepper, until they are well-coated. Set up the potatoes in the air fryer basket.
2. Bake on 360 F for 25 minutes, shaking once during cooking until crispy on the outside and tender on the inside. Serve warm.

Nutrition: Calories: 100 Carbs: 8 g Fat: 4 g Protein: 7 g

Homemade Peanut Corn Nuts

Preparation Time: 5 minutes

Cooking Time: 20 minutes

Servings: 4

Ingredients:

- 6 oz. dried hominy, soaked overnight
- 3 tbsp. peanut oil
- 2 tbsp. old bay seasoning
- Salt to taste

Directions:

1. Pat dry hominy and season with salt and old bay seasoning. Drizzle with oil and toss to coat. Spread in the air fryer basket and Air Fry for 10-12 minutes. Remove to shake up and return to cook for 10 more minutes until crispy. Transfer to a towel-lined plate to soak up the excess fat. Let cool and serve.

Nutrition: Calories: 100 Carbs: 3 g Fat: 3 g Protein: 5 g

Corn-Crusted Chicken Tenders

Preparation Time: 5 minutes

Cooking Time: 15 minutes

Servings: 4

Ingredients:

- 2 chicken breasts, cut into strips
- Salt and black pepper to taste
- 2 eggs
- 1 cup ground cornmeal

Directions:

1. In a bowl, mix ground cornmeal, salt, and black pepper. In another bowl, beat the eggs season with salt and pepper. Dip the chicken in the eggs and then coat in cornmeal. Spray the sticks with cooking spray and place them in the air fryer basket in a single layer. Air Fry for 6 minutes, slide the basket out and flip the sticks cook for 6-8 more minutes until golden brown.

Nutrition: Calories: 170 Carbs: 8 g Fat: 6 g Protein: 16 g

Choco Hazelnut Croissant

Preparation Time:15 minutes

Cooking Time: 10 minutes

Servings: 2

Ingredients:

- 1 oz. canned crescent rolls
- 8 teaspoons chocolate hazelnut spread

Directions:

1. Separate crescent dough into triangles.
2. Spread top with chocolate hazelnut spread.
3. Roll up the triangles to form a crescent shape.
4. Place these in the air fryer.
5. Select bake setting.
6. Cook at 320 degrees F for 8 to 10 minutes or until golden.

Nutrition: Calories 101 Fat 8.9 g Carbohydrates 3.6 g Sugar 0.5 g Protein 3.2 g Cholesterol 60 mg

Blueberry Muffin Surprise

Preparation Time:10 minutes

Cooking Time: 20 minutes

Servings:12

Ingredients:

- 2 eggs
- 1/2 tsp vanilla
- 1/2 cups Swerve
- 16 oz cream cheese
- 1/4 cup almonds, sliced
- 1/4 cup blueberries

Directions:

1. Preheat the cosori air fryer to 350 F.
2. In a mixing bowl, beat cream cheese until smooth.
3. Add eggs, vanilla, and sweetener and beat until well combined.
4. Add almonds and blueberries and fold well.
5. Spoon mixture into the silicone muffin molds.
6. Place molds in the air fryer basket and cook for 20 minutes. Cook in batches.

Nutrition: Calories 156 Fat 14.9 g Carbohydrates 2 g

Sugar 0.5 g Protein 4.2 g Cholesterol 69 mg

Blueberry Crumble

Preparation Time:15 minutes

Cooking Time: 15 minutes

Servings: 4

Ingredients:

- ½ cup blueberries, sliced
- 1 apple, diced
- 2 tablespoons butter
- 2 tablespoons sugar
- ¼ cup rice flour
- ½ teaspoon cinnamon powder

Directions:

1. Mix all the ingredients in a small baking pan.
2. Place inside the air fryer.
3. Choose bake setting.
4. Set it to 350 degrees F.
5. Cook for 15 minutes.

Nutrition: Calories 93 Fat 8.8 g Carbohydrates 1 g Sugar 0.2 g Protein 2.8 g Cholesterol 58 mg

Golden Caramelized Pear Tart

Preparation Time: 15 minutes

Cooking Time: 25 minutes

Serves 8

Ingredients:

- Juice of 1 lemon
- 4 cups water
- 3 medium or 2 large ripe or almost ripe pears (preferably Bosc or Anjou), peeled, stemmed, and halved lengthwise
- 1 sheet (½ package) frozen puff pastry, thawed
- All-purpose flour, for dusting
- 4 tablespoons caramel sauce such as Smucker's Salted Caramel, divided

Directions:

1. Combine the lemon juice and water in a large bowl.
2. Remove the seeds from the pears with a melon baller and cut out the blossom end. Remove any tough fibers between the stem

end and the center. As you work, place the pear halves in the acidulated water.

3. On a lightly floured cutting board, unwrap and unfold the puff pastry, roll it very lightly with a rolling pin so as to press the folds together. Place it on the sheet pan.

4. Roll about ½ inch of the pastry edges up to form a ridge around the perimeter. Crimp the corners together so as to create a solid rim around the pastry to hold in the liquid as the tart cooks.

5. Brush 2 tablespoons of caramel sauce over the bottom of the pastry.

6. Remove the pear halves from the water and blot off any remaining water with paper towels.

7. Place one of the halves on the board cut-side down and cut ¼-inch-thick slices radially. Repeat with the remaining halves. Arrange the pear slices over the pastry. Drizzle the remaining 2 tablespoons of caramel sauce over the top.

8. Place the basket on the bake position.

9. Select Bake, set temperature to 350ºF (180ºC), and set Time to 25 minutes.

10. After 15 minutes, check the tart, rotating the pan if the crust is not browning evenly. Continue cooking for another 10 minutes, or until the pastry is golden brown, the pears are soft, and the caramel is bubbling.

11. When done, remove the pan from the air fryer grill and allow to cool for about 10 minutes.

12. Served warm.

Nutrition: Calories 83 Fat 7.8 g Carbohydrates 1 g Sugar 0.3g Protein 2.9 g Cholesterol 58 mg

Middle East Baklava

Preparation Time: 10 minutes

Cooking Time: 16 minutes

Serves 10

Ingredients:

- 1 cup walnut pieces
- 1 cup shelled raw pistachios
- ½ cup unsalted butter, melted
- ¼ cup plus 2 tablespoons honey, divided
- 3 tablespoons granulated sugar
- 1 teaspoon ground cinnamon
- 2 (1.9-ounce) packages frozen miniature phyllo tart shells

Directions:

1. Place the walnuts and pistachios in the air fry basket in an even layer.
2. Place the basket on the air fry position.
3. Select Air Fry, set the temperature to 350ºF (180ºC), and set the Time for 4 minutes.
4. After 2 minutes, remove the basket and stir the nuts. Transfer the basket back to the air fryer grill and cook for another 1 to 2

minutes until the nuts are golden brown and fragrant.

5. Meanwhile, stir together the butter, sugar, cinnamon, and ¼ cup of honey in a medium bowl.

6. When done, remove the basket from the air fryer grill and place the nuts on a cutting board and allow to cool for 5minutes. Finely chop the nuts. Add the chopped nuts and all the "nut dust" to the butter mixture and stir well.

7. Arrange the phyllo cups on the basket. Evenly fill the phyllo cups with the nut mixture, mounding it up. As you work, stir the nuts in the bowl frequently so that the syrup is evenly distributed throughout the filling.

8. Place the basket on the bake position.

9. Select Bake, set temperature to 350ºF (180ºC), and set Time to 12 minutes. After about 8 minutes, check the cups. Continue cooking until the cups are golden brown and the syrup is bubbling.

10. When cooking is complete, remove the baklava from the air fryer grill, drizzle each cup with about 1/8teaspoon of the remaining honey over the top.

11. Allow to cool for 5 minutes before serving.

Nutrition: Calories 95 Fat 7.8 g Carbohydrates 2 g Sugar 0.2 g Protein 3.8 g Cholesterol 50 mg

Chocolate Donuts

Preparation Time:5 minutes

Cooking Time: 20 minutes

Servings: 8-10

Ingredients:

- (8-ounce) can jumbo biscuits
- cooking oil
- chocolate sauce, such as Hershey's
- Directions:
- Separate the biscuit dough into 8 biscuits and place them on a flat work surface. Use a small circle cookie cutter or a biscuit cutter to cut a hole in each biscuit center. You can also cut the holes using a knife.
- Grease the basket with cooking oil.
- Place 4 donuts in the air fryer oven. Do not stack. Spray with cooking oil. Cook for 4 minutes.
- Open the air fryer and flip the donuts. Cook for an additional 4 minutes.
- Remove the cooked donuts from the air fryer oven, then repeat for the remaining 4 donuts.

- Drizzle chocolate sauce over the donuts and enjoy while warm.

Nutrition: Calories: 181 protein: 3 g. Fat: 98 g. Carbs: 42 g.

Coconut Pancake

Preparation Time: 10 Minutes

Cooking Time: 20 Minutes

Servings: 4

Ingredients:

- 2 cups self-rising flour
- 2 tablespoons sugar
- 2 eggs
- 1 and 1/2 cups coconut milk
- A drizzle of olive oil

Directions:

1. In a bowl, mix eggs with sugar, milk, flour, and whisk until you obtain a batter.
2. Grease your air fryer with the oil, add the batter, spread into the pot, cover and cook on Low for 20 minutes.
3. Slice pancake, divide between plates and serve cold.

Nutrition: Calories: 162 Protein: 8 g. Fat: 3 g. Carbs: 7 g.

Cinnamon Rolls

Preparation Time: 2 Hours

Cooking Time: 15 Minutes

Servings: 8

Ingredients:

- 1-pound vegan bread dough
- ¾ cup coconut sugar
- 1 and 1/2 tablespoons cinnamon powder
- 2tablespoons vegetable oil

Directions:

1. Roll dough on a floured working surface, shape a rectangle and brush with the oil.
2. In a bowl, mix cinnamon with sugar, stir, sprinkle this over dough, roll into a log, seal well and cut into 8 pieces.
3. Leave rolls to rise for 2 hours, place them in your air fryer's basket, cook at 350 degrees F for 5 minutes, flip them, cook for 4 minutes more and transfer to a platter.
4. Enjoy!

Nutrition: Calories: 170 Protein: 6 g. Fat: 1 g. Carbs: 7 g.

Mixed Berries Crisp

Preparation Time:10 Minutes

Cooking Time: 12 Minutes

Serves 4

Ingredients:

- 1/2cup fresh blueberries
- 1/2cup chopped fresh strawberries
- 1/3cup frozen raspberries, thawed
- 1 tablespoon honey
- 1 tablespoon freshly squeezed lemon juice
- 2/3 cup whole-wheat pastry flour
- 3 tablespoons packed brown sugar
- 2 tablespoons unsalted butter, melted

Directions:

1. Place the strawberries, blueberries, and raspberries in a baking pan and drizzle the honey and lemon juice over the top.
2. Combine the pastry flour and brown sugar in a small mixing bowl.
3. Add the butter and whisk until the mixture is crumbly. Scatter the flour mixture on top of the fruit.
4. Place the pan on the bake position.

5. Set Time to 12 minutes.

6. When cooking is complete, the fruit should be bubbly and the topping should be golden brown.

Nutrition: Calories: 170 Carbs: 8 g Fat: 6 g Protein: 16 g

Duck Fat Roasted Red Potatoes

Preparation Time:5 minutes

Cooking Time: 25 minutes

Servings: 4

Ingredients:

- 4 red potatoes, cut into wedges
- 1 tbsp. garlic powder
- 2 tbsp. thyme, chopped
- 3 tbsp. duck fat, melted

Directions:

1. Preheat air fryer to 380 F. In a bowl, mix duck fat, garlic powder, salt, and pepper. Add the potatoes and shake to coat.
2. Place in the basket and bake for 12 minutes, remove the basket, shake and continue cooking for another 8-10 minutes until golden brown. Serve warm topped with thyme.

Nutrition: Calories: 110 Carbs: 8 g Fat: 5 g Protein: 7 g

Chicken Wings with Alfredo Sauce

Preparation Time:5 minutes

Cooking Time: 20 minutes

Servings: 4

Ingredients:

- 1 1/2 lb. chicken wings, pat-dried
- Salt to taste
- 1/2 cup Alfredo sauce

Directions:

1. Season the wings with salt. Arrange them in the greased air fryer basket, without touching and Air Fry for 12 minutes until no longer pink in the center. Work in batches if needed. Flip them, increase the heat to 390 F and cook for 5 more minutes. Plate the wings and drizzle with Alfredo sauce to serve.

Nutrition: Calories: 150 Carbs: 7 g Fat: 5 g Protein: 14 g

Crispy Squash

Preparation Time:5 minutes

Cooking Time: 20 minutes

Servings: 4

Ingredients:

- 2 cups butternut squash, cubed
- 2 tbsp. olive oil
- Salt and black pepper to taste
- ¼ tsp. dried thyme
- 1 tbsp. fresh parsley, finely chopped

Directions:

1. In a bowl, add squash, olive oil, salt, pepper, thyme, and toss to coat.
2. Place the squash in the air fryer and Air Fry for 14 minutes at 360 F, shaking once or twice. Serve sprinkled with fresh parsley.

Nutrition: Calories: 100 Carbs: 5 g Fat: 2 g Protein: 3 g

Classic French Fries

Preparation Time:5 minutes

Cooking Time: 30 minutes

Servings: 4

Ingredients:(2 servings)

- 2 russet potatoes, cut into strips
- 2 tbsp. olive oil
- Kosher salt and black pepper to taste
- 1/2 cup aioli

Directions:

1. Preheat the fryer to 400 F. Spray the air fryer basket with cooking spray.
2. In a bowl, brush the strips with olive oil and season with salt and black pepper. Put it in the air fryer and cook for 20-22 minutes, turning once halfway through, until crispy. Serve with garlic aioli.

Nutrition: Calories: 120 Carbs: 7 g Fat: 4 g Protein: 6 g

BBQ Chicken

Preparation Time:5 minutes

Cooking Time: 30 minutes

Servings: 4

Ingredients:

- 1 whole small chicken, cut into pieces
- 1 tsp. salt
- 1 tsp. smoked paprika
- 1 tsp. garlic powder
- 1 cup BBQ sauce

Directions:

1. Mix salt, paprika, and garlic powder and coat the chicken pieces. Place in the air fryer basket and Bake for 18 minutes at 400 F. Remove to a plate and brush with barbecue sauce.
2. Wipe the fryer clean from the chicken fat. Return the chicken to the fryer, skin-side up, and Bake for 5 more minutes at 340 F.

Nutrition: Calories: 230 Carbs: 12 g Fat: 9 g Protein: 23 g

Turkey Meatballs with Spaghetti Squash

Preparation Time: 15 minutes

Cooking Time: 35 minutes

Servings: 4

Ingredients:

- 1 lb. lean ground turkey
- 1 lb. spaghetti squash, halved and seeds removed
- 2 egg whites
- 1/3 cup green onions, diced fine
- ¼ cup onion, diced fine
- 2 ½ tbsp. flat leaf parsley, diced fine
- 1 tbsp. fresh basil, diced fine
- What you'll need from store cupboard:
- 14 oz. can no-salt-added tomatoes, crushed
- 1/3 cup soft whole wheat bread crumbs
- ¼ cup low sodium chicken broth
- 1 tsp garlic powder
- 1 tsp thyme
- 1 tsp oregano
- ½ tsp red pepper flakes

- ½ tsp whole fennel seeds

Directions:

1. In a small bowl, combine bread crumbs, onion, garlic, parsley, pepper flakes, thyme, and fennel.

2. In a large bowl, combine turkey and egg whites. Add bread crumb mixture and mix well. Cover and chill 10 minutes. Heat the oven to broil.

3. Place the squash, cut side down, in a glass baking dish. Add 3-4 tablespoons of water and microwave on high 10-12 minutes, or until fork tender.

4. Make 20 meatballs from the turkey mixture and place on a baking sheet. Broil 4-5 minutes, turn and cook 4 more minutes.

5. In a large skillet, combine tomatoes and broth and bring to a simmer over low heat. Add meatballs, oregano, basil, and green onions. Cook, stirring occasionally, 10 minutes or until heated through.

6. Use a fork to scrape the squash into "strands" and arrange on a serving platter. Top with meatballs and sauce and serve.

Nutrition: Calories 253 Total Carbs 15g Net Carbs 13g Protein 27g Fat 9g Sugar 4g Fiber 2g

Turkey & Mushroom Casserole

Preparation Time:15 minutes

Cooking Time: 50 minutes

Servings: 8

Ingredients:

- 1 lb. cremini mushrooms, washed and sliced
- 1 onion, diced
- 6 cup cauliflower, grated
- 4 cup turkey, cooked and cut in bite size pieces
- 2 cup reduced fat Mozzarella, grated, divided
- 1 cup fat free sour cream
- ½ cup lite mayonnaise
- ¼ cup reduced fat parmesan cheese
- 2 tbsp. olive oil, divided
- 2 tbsp. Dijon mustard
- 1 ½ tsp thyme
- 1 ½ tsp poultry seasoning

Directions:

1. Heat oven to 375 degrees. Spray a 9x13-inch baking dish with cooking spray.

2. In a medium bowl, stir together sour cream, mayonnaise, mustard, ½ teaspoon each thyme and poultry seasoning, 1 cup of the mozzarella, and parmesan cheese.

3. Heat 2 teaspoons oil in a large skillet over med-high heat. Add mushrooms and sauté until they start to brown and all liquid is evaporated. Transfer them to the baking dish.

4. Add 2 more teaspoons oil to the skillet along with the onion and sauté until soft and they start to brown. Add the onions to the mushrooms.

5. Add another 2 teaspoons oil to the skillet with the cauliflower. Cook, stirring frequently, until it starts to get soft, about 3-4 minutes. Add the remaining thyme and poultry seasoning and cook 1 more minute.

6. Season with salt and pepper and add to baking dish. Place the turkey over the vegetables and stir everything together.

7. Spread the sauce mixture over the top and stir to combine. Sprinkle the remaining mozzarella over the top and bake 40 minutes, or until bubbly and cheese is golden brown. Let cool 5 minutes, then cut and serve.

Nutrition: Calories 351 Total Carbs 13g Net Carbs 10g Protein 37g Fat 16g Sugar 5g Fiber 3g

Prosciutto-Wrapped Asparagus

Preparation Time:10 m

Cooking Time 12 m

6 Servings

Ingredients:

- 12 spears asparagus, trimmed
- 2 teaspoons olive oil
- Salt and freshly ground black pepper, to taste
- 12 prosciutto slices

Directions:

1. Drizzle the asparagus spears with oil and ten, sprinkle with salt and black pepper.
2. Wrap one prosciutto slice around each asparagus spear from top to bottom.
3. Turn the "Temperature Knob" of Power XL Air Fryer Grill to line the temperature to 300 degrees F.
4. Turn the "Function Knob" to settle on "Air Fry."
5. Turn the "Timer Knob" to line the Time for 10 minutes.

6. After preheating, arrange the asparagus spears into the greased air fry basket.
7. Insert the air fry basket at position 2 of the Air Fryer Grill.
8. Flip the asparagus spears once halfway through.
9. When the cooking Time is over, transfer the asparagus spears onto a platter.
10. Serve hot.

Nutrition: Calories: 144 Kcal, Fat: 8.7g, Carb: 1.9g, Protein: 16g

Coconut Shrimp

Preparation Time:15 m

Cooking Time 8 m

3 Servings

Ingredients:

- ¼ cup almond flour
- ½ teaspoon garlic powder, divided
- ½ teaspoon paprika, divided
- Salt and freshly ground black pepper, to taste
- 2 large eggs, beaten
- 1 tablespoon unsweetened almond milk
- ½ cup unsweetened flaked coconut
- ¼ cup pork rinds, crushed
- ½ pound large shrimp, peeled and deveined
- Nonstick cooking spray

Directions:

1. Place the flour, half the spices, salt, and black pepper in a shallow dish and blend well.
2. Place the eggs and almond milk in a second shallow dish and beat well.

3. Place the coconut, pork rinds, remaining spices, salt, and black pepper and blend well.

4. Coat shrimp with flour mixture, then read egg mixture and eventually coat with the coconut mixture.

5. 5 Again, dip in the egg mixture and coat with the coconut mixture.

6. 6 Turn the "Temperature Knob" of Power XL Air Fryer Grill to line the temperature to 380 degrees F.

7. 7 Turn the "Function Knob" to settle on "Air Fry."

8. 8 Turn the "Timer Knob" to line the Time for 8 minutes.

9. 9 After preheating, arrange the shrimp into the greased air fry basket.

10. Insert the air fry basket at position 2 of the Air Fryer Grill.

11. Flip the shrimp once halfway through.

12. When the cooking Time is over, transfer the shrimp onto a platter.

13. Serve immediately.

Nutrition: Calories: 234 Kcal, Fat: 13.8g, Carb, 5.9g,

Protein: 20g

Rice Bites

Preparation Time:10 m

Cooking Time 10 m

4 Servings

Ingredients:

- 3 cups cooked risotto
- 1/3 cup Parmesan cheese, grated
- 1 egg, beaten
- 3 ounces mozzarella cheese, cubed
- ¾ cup breadcrumbs
- Directions:
- In a bowl, mix the risotto, Parmesan cheese, and egg.
- Make 20 equal-sized balls from the mixture.
- Insert a mozzarella cube in the center of every ball.
- With your fingers, smooth the risotto mixture to hide the mozzarella.
- In a shallow dish, add the breadcrumbs.
- Coat the balls with breadcrumbs.
- Turn the "Temperature Knob" of Power XL Air Fryer Grill to line the temperature to 390 degrees F.

- Turn the "Function Knob" to settle on "Air Fry."
- Turn the "Timer Knob" to line the Time for 10 minutes.
- After preheating, arrange the balls in the air fryer basket in a single layer.
- Insert the air fryer basket at position 2 of the Air Fryer Grill.
- When the cooking Time is over, transfer the balls onto a platter.
- Serve warm.

Nutrition: Calories: 241 Kcal, Fat: 5.2g, Carb, 36.9g, Protein: 10g

Grilled Tomato Salsa

Preparation Time:15 Minutes

Cooking Time: 10 Minutes

Servings: 4 to 8

Ingredients:

- 1 onion, sliced
- 1 jalapeño pepper, sliced in half
- 5 tomatoes, sliced
- 2 tablespoons oil
- Salt and pepper to taste
- 1 cup cilantro, trimmed and sliced
- 1 tablespoon lime juice
- 1 teaspoon lime zest
- 2 tablespoons ground cumin
- 3 cloves garlic, peeled and sliced

Directions:

1. Coat onion, jalapeño pepper and tomatoes with oil.
2. Season with salt and pepper.
3. Add grill grate to your Power XL Grill.
4. Press grill setting.
5. Choose max temperature and set it to 10 minutes.

6. Press start to preheat.

7. Add vegetables on the grill.

8. Cook for 5 minutes per side.

9. Transfer to a plate and let cool.

10. Add vegetable mixture to a food processor.

11. Stir in remaining ingredients.

12. Pulse until smooth.

Nutrition: Calories - 369 Fat – 16g Carbohydrates – 37g Fiber – 5g Protein – 14g

Parmesan French Fries

Preparation Time:15 Minutes

Cooking Time: 15 Minutes

Servings: 6

Ingredients:

- 1 lb. French fries
- 1/2 cup mayonnaise
- 2 cloves garlic, minced
- 1 tablespoon oil
- Salt and pepper to taste
- 1 teaspoon garlic powder
- 1/2 cup Parmesan cheese, grated
- 1 teaspoon lemon juice

Directions:

1. Add crisper basket to your Power XL Grill.
2. Select air fry function.
3. Set it to 375 degrees F for 22 minutes.
4. Press start to preheat.
5. Add fries to the basket.
6. Cook for 10 minutes.
7. Shake and cook for another 5 minutes.
8. Toss in oil and sprinkle with Parmesan cheese.

9. Mix the remaining ingredients in a bowl.

10.   Serve fries with this sauce.

Nutrition: Calories - 445 Fat – 27g Carbohydrates –
25g Fiber – 2g Protein – 20g

Fish Sticks

Preparation Time:15 Minutes

Cooking Time: 15 Minutes

Servings: 8

Ingredients:

- 16 oz. tilapia fillets, sliced into strips
- 1 cup all-purpose flour
- 2 eggs
- 1 1/2 cups breadcrumbs
- Salt to taste

Directions:

1. Dip fish strips in flour and then in eggs.
2. Mix breadcrumbs and salt.
3. Coat fish strips with breadcrumbs.
4. Add fish strips to a crisper plate.
5. Place crisper plate inside the basket.
6. Choose air fry setting.
7. Cook fish strips at 390 degrees F for 12 to 15 minutes, flipping once halfway through.

Nutrition: Calories: 324 Fat: 21.5g Saturated Fat: 4g Trans Fat: 0g Carbohydrates: 7.5g Fiber: 2g Sodium: 274mg Protein: 20g

Homemade Fries

Preparation Time:15 Minutes

Cooking Time: 45 Minutes

Servings: 6

Ingredients:

- 1 lb. large potatoes, sliced into strips
- 2 tablespoons vegetable oil
- Salt to taste

Directions:

1. Toss potato strips in oil.
2. Add crisper plate to the air fryer basket inside the Power XL Grill.
3. Choose air fry function. Set it to 390 degrees F for 3 minutes.
4. Press start to preheat.
5. Add potato strips to the crisper plate.
6. Cook for 25 minutes.
7. Stir and cook for another 20 minutes.

Nutrition: Calories - 183 Fat, – 7.4g Carbohydrates – 5.4g Fiber – 1g Protein – 22.3g

Fried Garlic Pickles

Preparation Time: 20 Minutes

Cooking Time: 15 Minutes

Servings: 6

Ingredients:

- 1/4 cup all-purpose flour
- Pinch baking powder
- 2 tablespoons water
- Salt to taste
- 20 dill pickle slices
- 2 tablespoons cornstarch
- 1 1/2 cups panko bread crumbs
- 2 teaspoons garlic powder
- 2 tablespoons canola oil

Directions:

1. In a bowl, combine flour, baking powder, water and salt.
2. Add more water if batter is too thick.
3. Put the cornstarch in a second bowl, and mix breadcrumbs and garlic powder in a third bowl.

4. Dip pickles in cornstarch, then in the batter and finally dredge with breadcrumb mixture.
5. Add crisper plate to the air fryer basket inside the Power XL Grill.
6. Press air fry setting.
7. Set it to 360 degrees F for 3 minutes.
8. Press start to preheat.
9. Add pickles to the crisper plate.
10. Brush with oil.
11. Air fry for 10 minutes.
12. Flip, brush with oil and cook for another 5 minutes.

Nutrition: Calories - 112 Fat – 4.6g Carbohydrates – 18.6g Fiber – 2g Protein – 1.7g

Zucchini Strips with Marinara Dip

Preparation Time:1 Hour and 10 Minutes

Cooking Time: 30 Minutes

Servings: 8

Ingredients:

- 2 zucchinis, sliced into strips
- Salt to taste
- 1 1/2 cups all-purpose flour
- 2 eggs, beaten
- 2 cups bread crumbs
- 2 teaspoons onion powder
- 1 tablespoon garlic powder
- 1/4 cup Parmesan cheese, grated
- 1/2 cup marinara sauce

Directions:

1. Season zucchini with salt.
2. Let sit for 15 minutes.
3. Pat dry with paper towels.
4. Add flour to a bowl.
5. Add eggs to another bowl.
6. Mix remaining ingredients except marinara sauce in a third bowl.

7. Dip zucchini strips in the first, second and third bowls.
8. Cover with foil and freeze for 45 minutes.
9. Add crisper plate to the air fryer basket inside the Power XL Grill.
10. Select air fry function.
11. Preheat to 360 degrees F for 3 minutes.
12. Add zucchini strips to the crisper plate.
13. Air fry for 20 minutes.
14. Flip and cook for another 10 minutes.
15. Serve with marinara dip.

Nutrition: Calories: 364 Fat: 35g Saturated Fat: 17g Trans Fat: 0g Carbohydrates: 8g Fiber: 1.5g Sodium: 291mg Protein: 8g

Greek Potatoes

Preparation Time: 20 Minutes

Cooking Time: 30 Minutes

Servings: 4

Ingredients:

- 1 lb. potatoes, sliced into wedges
- 2 tablespoons olive oil
- 1 teaspoon paprika
- 2 teaspoons dried oregano
- Salt and pepper to taste
- 1/4 cup onion, diced
- 2 tablespoons lemon juice
- 1 tomato, diced
- 1/4 cup black olives, sliced
- 1/2 cup feta cheese, crumbled

Directions:

1. Add crisper plate to the air fryer basket inside the Power XL Grill.
2. Choose air fry setting.
3. Set it to 390 degrees F.
4. Preheat for 3 minutes.
5. While preheating, toss potatoes in oil.

6. Sprinkle with paprika, oregano, salt and pepper.

7. Add potatoes to the crisper plate.

8. Air fry for 18 minutes.

9. Toss and cook for another 5 minutes.

10. Add onion and cook for 5 minutes.

11. Transfer to a bowl.

12. Stir in the rest of the ingredients.

Nutrition: Calories – 368 Fat – 24.2g Carbohydrates – 21g Fiber – 4.1g Protein – 17.6g

Ranch Chicken Fingers

Preparation Time:15 Minutes

Cooking Time: 20 Minutes

Servings: 4

Ingredients:

- 2 lb. chicken breast fillet, sliced into strips
- 1 tablespoon olive oil
- 1 oz. ranch dressing seasoning mix
- 4 cups breadcrumbs
- Salt to taste

Directions:

1. Coat chicken strips with olive oil.
2. Sprinkle all sides with ranch seasoning.
3. Cover with foil and refrigerate for 1 to 2 hours.
4. In a bowl, mix breadcrumbs and salt.
5. Dredge the chicken strips with seasoned breadcrumbs.
6. Add crisper plate to the air fryer basket inside the Power XL Grill.
7. Choose air fry setting.
8. Set it to 390 degrees F.
9. Preheat for 3 minutes.

10. Add chicken strips to the crisper plate.

11. Cook for 15 to 20 minutes, flipping halfway through.

Nutrition: Calories – 188 Fat – 3.2g Carbohydrates – 28.5g Fiber – 6.2g Protein – 29.4g

Lightning Source UK Ltd.
Milton Keynes UK
UKHW022023240621
386092UK00002BA/307